RESET YOUR GUT DIET

3 EASY STEPS TO CHANGE YOUR DIET FOR LONG-TERM WEIGHT LOSS

MASON FORD

Second Edition - October 2024

ISBN: 9798344901374 (paperback)

CONTENTS

SECTION III

PREFACE

It has been 2.5 years since I published the first edition of *Reset Your Gut Diet*, and I am deeply grateful for the feedback and support from so many readers. Your comments and feedback have been invaluable in shaping this second edition.

In response to your concerns and suggestions, I have expanded and refined the content to ensure the information is more comprehensive and easier to follow. You will find a complete new chapter on dairy alternatives that specifically addresses concerns raised by some readers of the first edition of this book.

Additionally, the chapter that discusses the science behind this diet has been expanded, delving deeper into topics I believe will enhance your understanding of gut health and its profound impact on your overall well-being. This chapter (5) starts on page 45. Every scientific study that is being referenced in this book, can be found in the References section starting on page 97.

I also wanted you to know that I mention a few specific products in this book. I do not get any incentives from mentioning these products. However, these products are important for this diet as similar products from other companies do not produce the same results.

One of the most significant updates in this edition is the inclusion of a discussion concerning GLP-1 medications for weight loss. This includes how these medications can fit into the framework of resetting the gut for optimal health. You'll also learn how repairing your gut's microbiome through this diet affects your body's hormones such as GLP-1.

It is my sincere hope that this second edition will continue to serve as a trusted resource for you on your journey to better health. Thank you for your continued support and for allowing me to be part of your journey.

With gratitude,

Mason Ford

DISCLAIMER

While the author of this book is trained in molecular biology and neuroscience, he is not a medical doctor. Over the last decade, the author has been writing for several health-related blogs owing to his interest and knowledge on herbal remedies. Thus, this book is based on personal observations of the food we eat every day. The recommendations and suggestions given in this book are for informational purposes only, and may help you have a more positive relationship with food. However, the recommendations given in this book are not to be interpreted as medical advice, neither are they to be used to diagnose or treat any disease. Please consult your healthcare provider before starting any weight loss program. Your health should be monitored by a qualified healthcare professional if you wish to

This book is dedicated to my wife Jean and my sons Luke and Jude, who have always supported me in everything that I do. You all are a great inspiration to me and you make me proud every day!

INTRODUCTION

Can Skinny People Get Fat?

You may have been struggling to lose weight for years. You may have tried all kinds of diets and all kinds of plans. You may have even tried pills, but the weight has still not come off. Well, it is not your fault. Despite the thousands of diet plans, sophisticated exercise equipment and gym memberships that have been increasing year in year out, we're still getting fatter.

As a result, you may have now come to the conclusion that diets don't work! And in reality, this may be true - most diets do not work. Diets don't address the real problem, which is too much sugar, too much trans-fats and too much processed foods; not to mention, fast food is cheaper than healthy food, which encourages its consumption.

Every day, we're being exposed to thousands of chemicals in our food and our environment. When I say that you can lose the weight and keep it off for years to come, you may feel a little bit skeptical; in your shoes, I would be too, but I have a plan.

This plan is not a typical traditional diet; rather, it is a plan that takes care of the root problem that keeps you from losing weight. This plan takes the types of food you eat, when you eat them and how often you eat them into consideration. Armed with this knowledge, you will be able to make the necessary changes to your diet in order for you to finally lose weight.

At some point, I was almost discouraged from writing this book, but I eventually did because I believe there is a lot of misinformation about dieting and weight loss out there. This was the driving force that compelled me to get my own story out there, and in the process, help other people.

I'm not a doctor, but I'm trained in molecular biology, genetics and neuroscience. Over the years, I've seen too many people struggle with their weight, and now I've come to the realization that what causes diets to fail is the type of food.

It's not your fault that you're not losing weight. I believe it's how food and diet industries operate these days that expose us to foods that are laden with chemicals, trans-fats, and sugar.

When I was a kid, I was considered too skinny. I was also really tall. My doctor warned my parents that I needed to eat more because my low weight could jeopardize my health in the future, so, my parents did everything possible to have me gain weight.

I had to eat hot cereals with butter and sugar, and mashed potatoes with lots of gravy. I also had to drink chocolate milk, but nothing really helped; I just didn't gain the weight.

When I was in college, I enjoyed late nights watching hard-to-find horror movies with my roommates. In my experience, I can say that binge-watching makes you really hungry, so the challenge that my roommates and I came up with was, *"who can come up with the most greasy snacks and not just buy it, but also eat it?"*

After a few months of hanging out with my roommates, watching late night horror movies, I realized that I had gained a lot of weight.

Fast forward 15 years, I became a young father, and I gained a tremendous amount of weight. This was mostly because of bad eating habits: eating what my kids didn't finish, and ordering takeout several times a week.

This brings us to the question, are skinny people just lucky, and never get fat no matter what they eat? No, skinny people can get fat if they eat too much and make the wrong food choices.

As is documented in the documentary *"Supersize Me,"* the director, Morgan Spurlock ate only McDonald's food for 30 days. After consuming 5,000 calories a day (breakfast, lunch and dinner), he gained 24 lbs and experienced a number of health issues, including mood swings, a fatty liver and high cholesterol.

The reality TV series *"Fit to Fat to Fit"* shows what happens when healthy, fit personal trainers follow an extremely unhealthy diet and refrain from any exercise. Their goal was to better understand their clients, who were struggling with being overweight.

The show clearly shows the emotional toll of being overweight. As these trainers slowly became more obese, they became depressed, increased their blood pressure, became pre-diabetic and lost all their energy.

As my kids were getting older, I decided I wanted to live a healthier life, so I started to take a closer look at what I was eating on a daily basis. I was shocked at how much sugar, sodas and processed food I was consuming. I also realized that I did not eat enough protein; instead, I was eating too many carbs.

With that realization in mind, I made a few changes to my diet. I cut out all the bad stuff and added a few new items to my diet. Some of the items that I added to my diet were not chosen on purpose, but were actually added by chance (more about this in the following chapters).

At some point, I started to notice that most of my belly fat started to disappear. I had less food cravings and more energy. In the end, I lost more than 10% of my body weight. My pant sizes were four sizes lower.

If you want to live a healthier life, get rid of extra pounds forever, feel better and have more energy, this book is for you. I promise that this plan will work for you. If you stick with the plan, you will lose belly fat, including fat in your waist and hip area. You will feel more energized, and your food cravings will decrease.

This is a very simple plan that anybody can follow, but don't be fooled by the simplicity; it will offer you a workable solution to get rid of body fat, lose the weight you want and keep it off forever.

Of course, you can jump right in and skip to the later chapters to find all the details of this plan, but that will beat the purpose of losing weight forever. You need to discover the data of **why you're not losing weight**, which will be covered in detail in the first couple chapters. With data comes power. The data will show you what has been holding you back for years.

You will have the power to overcome your weight challenge! You can tweak your diet with the changes that I'll describe in this book, and be on your way to a healthier you, with less body fat, more energy and less food cravings.

SECTION I

The Battle
With Food

1

NOT ANOTHER DIET...
WHAT YOU'RE NOT GETTING WITH THIS BOOK

The weight loss industry in America reached an all-time high of $78 billion in 2019. About half of all Americans attempt to lose weight through dieting. Every year, millions of people buy diet plans, as a New Year resolution. Just take a look at how many ads you'll see right after the New Year, promising that you'll lose 20, 30 pounds as long as you buy their meal plan, shakes or diet supplements.

These diets sell the false belief that you can lose weight simply by restricting calories and by starting an exercise program. These diets may work initially, because you may lose weight due to the loss of water and good fats that protect your organs.

The only real effect these diets have is to permanently lower your metabolism[1]. When you stop the diet, you will gain the weight back, and add some more. All these diets do is make you feel guilty about your food, lower your metabolism, increase food cravings, make you miserable, and cost you money.

How many times have you stopped a diet, only to realize you were still being charged a monthly fee nine months later?

With this book, this is what you're *not* getting:

- **A Restrictive Diet**: It's also known as counting calories or points (e.g., low-calorie diets). These types of diet involve counting calories or points. An example of this kind of diet is the popular *Weight Watchers* diet. Weight Watchers was founded in 1963, and has millions of members. Each person has a particular set of points tailored to his or her needs. Healthy foods such as vegetables, fruits and lean protein have zero points, and serve as an incentive to make healthier food choices, however, consuming food while counting calories or points feels unnatural. In the long run, it makes you feel bad and guilty about your food choices, and it will make you miserable. Counting calories or points only lowers your resting metabolism, and makes you gain even more weight and fat eventually.

- **A high protein diet** (for example, the Atkins Diet): The Atkins diet is a high fat, high protein and low-carbohydrate diet, which consists of 4 phases. The first phase involves eating less than 20 grams of carbohydrates each day for 2 weeks. During the second phase, nuts, vegetables and some fruits are added. In phase 3, more carbs are added to the diet until the weight loss slows down. The fourth phase is the maintenance phase which includes as many carbohydrates the body can handle without gaining weight. The Atkins diet is one of the most popular diets in history. This diet may work initially, but who wants to eat eggs, bacon and steak every day? If you're not careful, you'll eat non-organic meats and eggs, and actually disrupt your metabolism even more. More so, a high protein and high fat diet can raise your cholesterol levels; it is also very damaging to your liver, kidneys and heart in the long run.
- **A low-fat diet:** This diet involves lowering the percentage of fat in one's diet. Calorie intake is reduced because less fat is consumed. However, your body needs fats for healthy skin and hair, and for the production of hormones.

While a low-fat diet has been reported to result in weight loss, eliminating fats from your diet will lower your metabolism over longer periods of time, and does not address insulin resistance. Hence, this will eventually result in more weight gain. Also, it will take away the joy derived from eating.

- **The Mono Diet** (for example, the bread-only diet or salads): Nobody has ever lost weight permanently by eating one food or one food group. The bread-only diet has many side effects, because your body is missing out on essential nutrients such as vitamins, amino acids and fats. This can cause bad vision, lowered testosterone, weaker bones, and bad skin and hair. Eating salads to lose weight is another example of a mono diet. Unless you buy a well-balanced salad in a high-end restaurant, salads are kind of boring and do not always satisfy your hunger or provide enough nutritional benefits. If the lettuce used in the salad is not washed properly, potential *E. coli* contamination can make you really sick. Because salads don't have a high nutritional value and are often loaded with high-fat and high-calorie dressings, I don't think salads are a good way to lose weight. If you're looking to increase your fiber intake, you are better off eating regular vegetables that offer a higher nutritional benefit.

- **Meal kits:** Many expensive diets come packaged with meal kits, many of which are highly processed. Meal kits are heavily advertised by celebrities. They work in the short term by restricting calories, but because you're restricting calories over a period of many months, your metabolism will eventually slow down. That is why many people regain their weight as soon as they stop the diet. Many meal kits are heated by microwave, which kills many nutrients; they are loaded with chemicals. A highly popular diet that has been around for a few decades is the *Slimfast* diet. It consists of a shake for breakfast, a shake for lunch and a regular "sensible" dinner. But what is a "sensible" dinner? Another diet that uses meal kits is the Jenny Craig diet. The Jenny Craig diet has been popular since 1985. The idea was to help people make healthier food choices and wean them off the meal kits. A popular meal kit diet that is heavily targeted at men is Nutrisystem. Their plan offers breakfast, lunch and dinner for 5 days a week. It tries to appeal to men who desperately want to lose weight, but don't have the time to shop for their own food or have the motivation to change their eating habits. The problem with meal kits is that they are highly processed and contain many chemicals that slowly lower your metabolism. Most meal kits also don't teach customers how to develop healthy eating habits required to maintain the weight loss after stopping the diet plan.

- **Dietary supplements:** With the plan you're about to read (and will hopefully follow), there is no need for pills or dietary supplements. A popular dietary supplement that has been in the market for many years is Hydroxycut. Before 2004, Hydroxycut's main ingredient was ephedra. However, in 2004, the FDA banned the use of ephedra, which had been linked to 155 deaths from heart attacks and stroke. Hydroxycut was put back on the market without ephedra, but the maker of Hydroxycut was forced to recall their product in 2009, after the FDA received reports of liver problems, seizures and a muscle-wasting condition in some people who took the supplement. After 2009, the manufacturer changed the ingredients in Hydroxycut again; it now contains mainly caffeine and Robusta coffee extract.

- **Intermittent Fasting:** A review of a number of studies of intermittent fasting shows that it makes people lose weight. This form of weight loss is similar to weight loss from a calorie-restrictive diet. Intermittent fasting involves skipping either a day of eating or restricting your eating to just a specific period in a day. Although people do lose weight with this diet, it is difficult to maintain if you're a shift worker or have a busy job. It is still unclear if intermittent fasting has a negative influence on your metabolism in the long run.

With this book, my aim is to make you have a better sense of what you're eating every day. It's not a traditional diet, but something that I stumbled upon by accident. Over the years, this plan has proven to me that a particular combination of foods - which I will discuss later in the book - can lower your insulin resistance, lower your cravings for food and make you lose weight, especially the fat in specific areas. But first, we have to get a sense of what is holding you back and making you fat. And that will be covered in the next chapter.

2

WHY YOU'RE NOT LOSING WEIGHT

You may have tried a number of different diets in the past unsuccessfully, after eating too much during the holidays or hoping to lose some weight quickly before going on that dream trip. These type of diets have probably been successful at first, but now that you've stopped, you've gained the weight back, plus a few extra pounds.

It's not your fault. You do not need to feel guilty about your failed diet attempts. It's possible you don't eat too much, but have still been gaining weight as you grow older. At times, you find that even as you exercise, the weight never comes off.

The obesity rate in the United States has steadily increased during the last five decades. With new diet plans being introduced constantly, and millions of people dieting every year, you would think the obesity rates would eventually come down.

Even countries where obesity rates were historically low (such as countries in South-East Asia and South America) have seen obesity rates significantly rise after the introduction of fast food chains and processed foods.

Perhaps it's not so much how much we eat, but the *kind of foods* we eat. The foods we eat make us fat. Most non-organic foods are loaded with chemicals that have a negative effect on our organs, hormones and metabolism.

In this chapter, I will review the various hormones that regulate our hunger and satiety, and how ingredients and chemicals in our food influence the effectiveness and function of these hormones.

Insulin Effect on Weight

Insulin is a hormone secreted by the beta cells of the pancreas. The role of insulin is to inhibit food intake and to promote the use of carbohydrates for energy production.

Insulin levels increase after a meal, and cause carbo-hydrates to be used for energy. When insulin levels are low, the body uses mainly fats as an energy source.

Understanding how different foods affect the insulin response may be important for the treatment or the prevention of weight gain and diabetes.

Many studies have been done in the past that rank foods according to the extent in which they increase blood glucose levels. This is sometimes referred to as the Glycemic Index Factor, which is a ranking of foods based on their effect on blood sugar levels. Not every food has the same insulin response or GI factor.

Different foods containing the same amount of carbo-hydrate will not produce the same metabolic effect. Typical foods that have the highest insulin response are white bread, white rice, potatoes and candy. The foods that increase insulin the most however are, refined and processed foods.

Foods with the lowest insulin response are all-bran cereals, pasta, eggs, cheese and peanuts.

Protein-rich foods have the lowest glucose **and** insulin responses.

Meals that are high in fat and protein also have a low insulin response. For this reason, a high-fat/high-protein to carbohydrate ratio is ideal. We're not talking about avoiding foods that stimulate insulin, but rather, avoiding high-insulin-response foods in between meals.

The Effect of Fructose on Weight

Consumption of fructose from sugar and high-fructose corn syrup increased by 26% between 1970 and 1997.

High-fructose corn syrup was introduced to U.S. food manufacturing in the 1970s, mainly because of food subsidies, and it was adopted by the beverage industry in the 1980s to replace sugar as a sweetener.

The hormones - insulin and leptin - both regulate energy.

Insulin is secreted in response to high glucose levels in the blood. It promotes the burning of carbohydrates for energy, and the synthesis of proteins inside cells.

Leptin, on the other hand, is the hormone secreted by fat tissue and certain cells in the gut. It acts primarily on the brain, by **inhibiting** hunger.

However, fructose (as in high-fructose corn syrup) does not stimulate the pancreas to release insulin as regular sugar does. This is why you will experience a smaller insulin response if you consume a diet rich in fructose by drinking many sodas every day.

The hormone, leptin, is in turn stimulated by insulin. By consuming a large amount of fructose, you will also lower the leptin response.

Lowered insulin and leptin responses will result in increased food cravings and increased fat storage.

The end result of a lower insulin and leptin response over time, is increased weight gain and metabolic disease (which is hypertension, coronary artery disease and obesity).

More than 50% of men and women in the United States over the age of 20 are considered overweight with a BMI of more than 25. BMI, which stands for Body Mass Index, is a value derived from dividing your weight (in kilograms) by the square of your height (in meters). A BMI between 18.5 and 24.9 is considered normal weight. Nearly 25% of adults are clinically obese, with a BMI of more than 30.

The consumption of fructose has largely increased because of increased use of fructose in the production of sodas and other foods (candy, fast food, soda, packaged breakfast foods, condiments and blended juice drinks, just to name a few).

For example, just 2 twelve-ounce sodas contain up to 50 grams of fructose, or more than 10% of the energy requirements for an average weight woman.

Under **normal conditions**, the hormone insulin causes lower food intake and lower fat deposits.

However, there has been a misconception that insulin does the exact opposite. This misconception has led to the promotion of numerous diets, suggesting that weight loss can be achieved by avoiding foods that stimulate insulin secretion.

It's not the insulin secretion that's the problem, but the insulin *resistance* in the body.

Insulin resistance can be caused by consuming too much high-fructose corn syrup. High fructose levels in the blood increases the rate of fat production in the liver, and leads to insulin resistance.

Insulin resistance is the condition where insulin levels are increased, but insulin binding to the receptor is decreased, thereby limiting the effectiveness of insulin.

Recent studies have also identified people who have a problem with the hormone leptin. People with defects in the leptin receptor suffer from overeating and obesity.

Several recent animal studies have shown that over time, fructose consumption (as in high-fructose corn syrup) can result in insulin resistance: a reduced glucose response (not able to get rid of high sugar spikes in the blood), high levels of insulin, high blood pressure and increased fat deposits were all associated with fructose consumption in animal models.

The Problem with Fast Food

Fast food consumption has exploded in the last 30 years. Fast food is usually high in fat, high in saturated fat, is energy-dense, contains high-fructose corn syrup, and is low in fiber.

A typical fast food meal delivers 1,400 calories, which is 85% of the recommended daily fat intake and 73% of the recommended saturated fat intake.

Fast food is often paired with equally large portions of fructose-sweetened soft drinks, which further contribute to excessive energy intake.

Insulin resistance and excess insulin are more closely linked to saturated fats than unsaturated fats. A diet rich in saturated fat is a high predictor of developing insulin resistance.

Fast foods are **energy-dense foods**, which may interfere with the mechanisms that control our appetite.

We tend to ingest a similar bulk and weight of food every day. Consuming energy-dense foods will increase your daily caloric intake, and consuming fast foods regularly will increase the insulin response. The insulin response will stay high, even four to six hours after the food is consumed; this causes a low blood glucose level, which will make you feel hungry again, before your previous meal is even digested.

The high content of fructose in fast food and sodas, also has an effect on another appetite hormone called ghrelin.

Ghrelin is a hunger hormone that is secreted in the gut; it makes you feel hungry.

Mice that lack the hunger hormone ghrelin, eat less food, store less of their calories as fat, use more fat as energy and further accumulate less body weight than regular mice.

Ghrelin is not being suppressed when there's a lot of fructose in the bloodstream. This means that if you're consuming a large amount of high-fructose corn syrup each day, **you are constantly feeling hungry**.

Trans Fats Are Making You Fat

Trans fat is a type of unsaturated fat that naturally occurs in small amounts in breast milk and butter. However, the fast food industry and other industries have used large amounts of *partially hydrogenated* trans fat in many food products for a number of reasons.

To produce partially hydrogenated fats, liquid oils (unsaturated) are heated in the presence of hydrogen.

This hydrogenation process converts some of the unsaturated fatty acids into saturated fatty acids, which then turns the oil into solid fat, and increases its melting point (this process turns oils into shortening).

Trans fats are more resistant to oxidation, and therefore, have a longer shelf life.

Partially hydrogenated trans fats can be found in baked goods, fast foods and most snacks.

Trans fats have been linked to an increase in coronary artery disease in part by raising levels of bad cholesterol. It is for that reason that many cities, such as New York City, have banned the use of trans fats in restaurants.

For decades, we've been told that dietary fat is the main cause of obesity, and that we have to replace dietary fat with carbohydrates. However, many studies have proven quite the opposite - that dietary fat does not contribute to increased weight gain, and trans fats in our diets are the primary factors responsible for obesity and insulin resistance!

There has been a recent study on the effect of trans fats on the health of monkeys. Two groups of monkeys, who were fed the same calories each day, were studied. One group was receiving a regular fat diet, while the other group was receiving a diet rich in trans fats. After six years, monkeys who were on the trans-fat diet gained more weight with more abdominal fat deposits, increased insulin and insulin resistance.

Another study looked at the effects of trans fats and high-fructose corn syrup in mice. Mice were either fed a regular diet or a diet high in trans fats and high-fructose corn syrup. The study concluded that trans fats in the diet led to fatty liver disease and obesity. Furthermore, the addition of high-fructose corn syrup in the diet of some of these mice led to increased food consumption and insulin resistance.

In the last few decades, what has happened with our food is that we've been told over and over again to replace fats in our diets with carbohydrates.

At the same time, food manufacturers have been producing thousands of low-fat foods that have the same energy density as the original, more fatty food. The difference is that most of the fat has been replaced by sugar.

Since trans fats have been linked to obesity, inflammation, fatty liver disease, and weight gain, it is important to replace trans fats and hydrogenated fats in our diet with non-hydrogenated, unsaturated fats, such as olive oil and avocado oil.

Hence, we shouldn't just focus on fat intake alone, but focus more on **total** energy intake and physical activity.

Energy that we gain from food is expressed in calories, as is the energy burned when we exercise.

High-energy-dense foods (i.e., pizza, bread, candy) provide more energy per gram of food than lower-energy-dense foods (i.e., dairy, vegetables).

In order to lose weight properly and make it sustainable, we should focus on reductions in *energy-density* rather than focusing on replacing fats with carbohydrates.

Effects of Pesticides on Metabolism

An alternative reason why there is an obesity epidemic is the way our food is being produced - the use of drugs and chemicals in industrial farming of both animals and vegetables, as well as in the processing and packaging of these foods. These include pesticides, herbicides, hormones, food additives and plasticizers. Herbicides and pesticides in non-organic food have a negative impact on metabolism, and they disrupt insulin signaling.

BPA, also known as Bisphenol A, is a chemical, commonly used in food and beverage containers. It is a potential cause of diabetes and insulin resistance.

BPA is a compound that can be considered a weak

estrogen, based on its low binding affinity to the estrogen receptors.

Several animal studies have shown that BPA can interfere with hormonal signaling pathways, and cause a lower beta cell function in the pancreas, so that less insulin is being produced.

There are many pesticides (organophosphates and carbamates) used in farming and gardening that are highly neurotoxic, disrupting both male and female hormones, and showing a negative effect on sugar and fat metabolism.

It is believed that these pesticides also inhibit the enzyme acetylcholinesterase, which breaks down the neurotransmitter acetylcholine.

A build-up of acetylcholine disrupts normal neuro-transmission, and affects the peripheral and central nervous systems, muscles, liver, pancreas and the brain.

Several studies have reported that chronic exposure to these pesticides are linked to diabetes or other metabolic disorders. For example, the pesticide, Malathion, which you can buy at many home improvement and garden centers, has been linked to increased blood sugar and insulin levels.

Hormonal Imbalance Causing Weight Gain

Many studies have been done to study the effects of hormonal imbalance on weight gain. Studies on the effect of reduced levels of estrogen in menopausal women have concluded that less estrogen does not result in weight gain per se, but does result in increased fat deposits in the central abdomen. Increased fat accumulation during menopause can be decreased by eating foods rich in estrogen.

Obesity in men is sometimes associated with reduced testosterone levels. Reduced total testosterone in men is linked to a number of conditions, including erectile dysfunction, gynecomastia ("man boobs"), cardiovascular disease and insulin resistance. Some studies suggest that treatment with androgens can sometimes improve these conditions, increasing lean muscle mass and lowering fat deposits.

An under-active thyroid gland - also known as hypothyroidism - can also cause weight gain. Thyroid hormones are important for your metabolism. When inadequate thyroid hormone is produced, you won't be able to lose weight when on a diet.

Other symptoms of hypothyroidism include fatigue, brittle nails, dry skin, sleepiness, depression, muscle cramps, joint pains, constipation and water retention. More than 5 million Americans suffer from thyroid issues, and many of them don't even know it. Thyroid disease is a serious health condition that should be treated by a healthcare professional.

Bad Eating Habits

There are some things we can take responsibility for: constantly snacking throughout the day results in an elevated insulin response and could lead to insulin resistance over time.

You may not even be aware of how often you snack throughout the day. Maybe you eat a few snacks every time you enter the kitchen, or you sit down with a bag of chips while you're binge-watching your favorite show.

Are you aware of how often you snack each day? Do you snack because you're hungry or do you snack because you're upset or feeling anxious?

With our extremely busy lifestyles, it's very tempting to say you're too busy or too tired to cook a healthy meal, and instead, grab some fast food.

Fast food is everywhere, but know that consuming fast food - which is loaded with hormones, pesticides, herbicides, and high-fructose corn syrup - will disrupt your metabolism, and leads to extreme weight gain.

A peculiar habit that many parents are guilty of is finishing their kids' dinner when they're dining at a restaurant. This is because most of them feel guilty about leaving food, or maybe they were raised with the "clean plate" mentality.

To stop this habit, you have to stop feeling guilty about wasting food. Your child chose the food and ate enough food to satisfy their hunger. Resist the urge to finish their food. You already ate your own dinner, so, there is no reason to add more calories to your diet by finishing your kids' dinner. You will promote healthy eating habits by showing them that enough is enough too!

In summary, what happens in our gut with its many digestive and hormonal processes, greatly impacts our overall health and how we feel.

The foods we eat every day determine how well the gut functions. Every day, more studies are published about how our gut regulates our appetite.

The fact that gastric bypass surgery in many cases can reverse diabetes raises the possibility of an unrecognized effect of the gut in the development of diabetes.

In the next couple of chapters, you'll learn which foods have a detrimental effect on the gut, and are prone to make you overweight, and how to greatly improve your gut's health to set you up for long-lasting weight loss.

SECTION II

Setting The Stage

3

A PLAN FOR CHANGE

HOW TO GET YOUR BODY READY FOR WEIGHT LOSS

Y ou may have struggled with your weight for a long time. You've probably made futile attempts with several diet plans in the past. As you've read in the previous chapters, most diet plans in the market don't really teach you how to make healthy food choices for long-term weight loss success. In addition, the meal plans that come with some of these diets are overly processed, low in nutrients and contain chemicals that will disrupt your metabolism.

The old concept of calories in, calories out, has been proven wrong. Most diet plans are still based on this decades-old math equation (e.g., calorie-restrictive diets or points diets).

Your weight and how many calories you burn each day are dependent on a number of factors. For example, the type and number of bacteria that are living in your gut have a great influence on how many calories are absorbed from your food.

Studies have shown that people who are thin have different micro-organisms living in their gut than those who are obese.

Your brain also determines how many calories you burn each day. This *"metabolism set-point"* is determined by your genes, your environment and your behavior.

Your brain does everything in its power to make sure that your weight does not go below this set point. That is another reason why it is so difficult for most people to lose weight: it takes a very long time to increase your metabolism.

In this chapter, I'm going to discuss how to become more aware of the foods you eat every day, in order to get your body ready for substantial weight loss. I'm not talking about starvation, but rather, replacing the calories you eat now with high protein, low-energy-dense foods.

Compared to high-energy foods, low-energy-dense foods provide less calories for the same amount of weight.

In the last chapter, we learned about the importance of the hormones insulin and leptin, and also about the importance of the gut in maintaining proper weight and body fat. The concept of keeping the insulin-leptin response balanced while feeding the good bacteria in the gut, will be addressed in this chapter.

How Many Calories Do You Need Each Day?

Many diets are solely based on restrictive calorie intake. They may work in reducing the number you see on your scale for a short time, however, at some point your weight plateaus. This is because restrictive calorie "diets" result in lean muscle loss.

Lean muscle tissue is key in burning fat. When you lose lean muscle tissue due to lack of calories, it lowers your metabolism, and in turn causes your body to store calories as fat vs. burning them. When your metabolism is lowered, you will stop losing weight. Once you stop the "dieting," you will gain the weight back and then some more! This is why restricting calories alone DOESN'T work, and keeps you on the diet yo-yo.

In order for this plan to work, you will need to become aware of the calories you consume every day - not just by number, but by the qualities they possess. You have to look out for qualities that lead to long-term weight loss. Once you know the amount and type of calories you consume each day, you will begin to make life-long changes.

The entire process of getting a clear picture of what you eat every day may take 4-6 weeks. For this, I suggest you use the app, Lose It! which is a free app from both the App Store and the Google Play Store. This app is not only great to get a hang of how many calories you consume every day, but will also allow you understand the optimal portion sizes to achieve your goal weight.

After you download the app, you will have to add some specifics about your height, weight and age. You can also add your goal weight to the app, or you could keep your weight the way it is.

If you do decide to lose weight, the optimal weight to lose per week is not more than two pounds per week, which is the most the app will allow. Anything over two pounds per week is unhealthy.

You will record every meal you eat, including snacks, for four to six weeks. This will be your food diary, and it is an essential part of this journey. Therefore, it's important that you are honest with yourself, and don't skip anything you eat.

If you have take-out food, you may find several different calorie counts in the app for the same food. For example, a hamburger could give you several results, anywhere from 380 to 710 calories. It's best to do a little research before recording. Most fast food restaurants have their own nutrition information on their website. If you eat out at a restaurant that does not have their nutritional information available, you may run the risk of undercounting your calories. As a practice, you should add 50% more calories to be closer to the actual amount. After you do this for a number of weeks, you'll start to realize the types of food you eat often, your typical portion sizes, and how much snacking you do throughout the day.

The first goal of this plan is to limit yourself to three regular meals a day; that is breakfast, lunch and dinner, plus two small snacks in between. The reason for this is, we want the insulin response to stay low between the meals, and only peak three times per day.

Eliminate Processed Foods and Sodas

The second goal of this plan is to have a **healthier gut**. In order to do this, you need to eliminate most of the processed and refined foods, and switch to a more organic food plan. I know organic foods are more expensive, but it will be worth it in the long run. If you shop at regular grocery stores most of the time, I would suggest considering shopping at Whole Foods or Trader Joe's, or even shopping at a farmer's market on the weekend.

As I explained in the previous chapter, non-organic foods are loaded with chemicals, hormones, pesticides and herbicides, which in the long run, mess with your metabolism.

Pay particular attention to foods that contain flour. Non-organic flour may contain traces of herbicides. The herbicide glyphosate, for example, is not only a neuro-toxin, but can also lower your metabolism.

Glyphosate inhibits the pathway in plants and bacteria that converts fructose into aromatic amino acids. By consuming non-organic foods that contain trace amounts of glyphosate, the good bacteria in your gut will not be able to break down fructose as well. The liver will then convert that extra fructose into fat.

You also want to look at the Lose It! app and identify how many times each day you consume foods that are high in gluten. Gluten is a protein found in flour that can cause inflammation in the gut, especially in a lot of people who are sensitive to the gluten protein.

Gluten is also a high-energy-dense food. As I will explain in the next chapter, your goal is to replace some of the gluten that's in your diet with alternative food that is similar in bulk and weight, high in protein and lower in energy.

The Lose It! app will also show you how many times a week you eat fast food. I don't have to tell you that fast food is bad for you. You want to make sure that you eliminate fast food as much as possible. This specifically includes the sodas that come with fast food. You really should eliminate anything that contains high-fructose corn syrup from your diet. This is not just sodas, but any food that contains high-fructose corn syrup. You'll be surprised how many foods contain high-fructose corn syrup. For example, something as innocent-looking as popular crackers contain high-fructose corn syrup.

You may also say, "Oh, I'll just replace my regular sodas with diet soda." But diet soda is not good for you either. It's loaded with chemicals, and the man-made chemical sweeteners will lower your metabolism in the long run.

If you're going to replace sodas with something else, look for seltzer water or anything with bubbles that doesn't contain any sugars, but instead, contains stevia or has natural flavoring.

This is not going to be easy, and it's not your fault. Losing weight is really hard. It's not just a matter of willpower. Right now, your gut is in control. An out-of-balance gut that has been fed processed foods, sugar, trans-fat and too much gluten is going to remind you all day long that it wants more - more sugar, more fat, more carbs! It's almost like having a monster living in your gut that calls the shots.

Another point to note is that your brain is programmed to preserve calories, and anything that changes its status quo is met with resistance. So, you may feel pretty crappy if you try to eliminate sodas or eliminate any energy-dense foods such as pizzas. But you have to take into consideration the end goal of this plan, which is to feel good about yourself and lose weight forever.

In summary, the goal of this phase is to get a hang of the foods you consume every day. You're going to be using the free app Lose It! and you'll have to record everything you eat for the next four to six weeks. You're going to identify problematic foods (fast food, processed food, sodas) and replace them with healthier organic foods.

You don't have to count calories forever, so, after four to six weeks, your brain will be trained to determine the correct portion size for your body.

In the next chapter, I will describe how to add just a few foods to your diet in order to maintain a **lower and more stable insulin response** throughout the day. This way, you will lose fat from your problem areas and lose weight for the foreseeable future.

4

THE SIMPLE DIET PLAN

I f you have taken the steps outlined in the previous chapter, you're in a good spot! You are now aware of the foods you're eating on a daily basis, and you now feel empowered enough to make the necessary changes to your diet, so you can finally lose the weight!

After six weeks of recording your food, you have a clear picture of what needs to be eliminated from your diet. After you have recorded your food for 4-6 weeks, you will begin to recognize patterns, as most people eat similar foods every week.

When you scroll through your food recordings in the Lose It! app, pay attention to processed foods, sodas and fast foods. These foods need to be eliminated from your diet if you want to see results. Also, try to identify so-called energy-dense foods such as pizza and hoagies or subs.

The next phase of this plan involves adding three foods to your diet; replacing three high-energy-dense foods with foods that are similar in bulk, but lower in energy.

Without getting into any specifics, these three foods include a probiotic drink, organic Greek yogurt and organic cheese as a snack.

These three foods combined will lower food cravings, and add good bacteria to your gut. The end result is a more balanced insulin response throughout the day, less hunger, more energy and weight loss.

You may wonder how I came up with these three foods? I actually stumbled on it by accident. It all started in 2012, when the *"Greek yogurt craze"* was happening. As a scientist, I wondered, *"Does this stuff really work?"* I started eating Greek yogurt a few times a week for lunch, and surprisingly, I started to lose weight. Around that same period, I was experiencing bloating in my abdomen. For that, I picked up a bottle of Kevita probiotic drink and started drinking Kevita two to three times a week.

As for the cheese, my young kids got it when they would often come to the grocery store with me. They were allowed to pick out one snack each. One day, they chose Babybel Cheese (Mini Babybel). After a few weeks, when the bag of Babybel Cheese was sitting unopened in the fridge, I figured I didn't want to throw it out, so I started eating it.

After a few weeks of eating Greek yogurt, drinking Kevita probiotic drinks and snacking on Babybel Cheese, I noticed that I was starting to lose weight, had less food cravings and had more energy throughout the day. The weight just kept coming off, until I was at a healthier weight.

One day, I thought, *"What will happen if I eliminate one of these three foods?"* So, first, I stopped snacking on the Babybel cheese, and some weight returned. Then I kept the Greek yogurt and Babybel cheese, and eliminated the Kevita probiotic drink. I noticed I gained some weight again! The same thing happened when I eliminated the Greek yogurt and kept the Babybel Cheese and the probiotic drink.

For some reason, the Greek yogurt, probiotic drink and Babybel Cheese work really well together in making you lose weight and suppress food cravings! Now, you know how it all started. And now, I'm ready to tell you the specifics of how to add these three food items to your diet.

Breakfast

For breakfast, eat one small cup of FAGE Greek yogurt (5.3 ounces serving size) combined with a cup of coffee (8-12 Oz.). Either 0% or 2% fat FAGE Greek yogurt will do, and it can also come plain or with fruit flavoring. Eat the Greek yogurt for breakfast four to five times per week. Sometimes, you may add an egg.

It is important to stick to the FAGE Greek yogurt and not be tempted to use other brands of Greek yogurt based on taste or price. It is *brand specific* - I have tried several other brands of Greek yogurts over the years, and none had the same effect on weight as FAGE yogurt. Furthermore, there are a few other Greek yogurts that use fillers such as modified food starch, which you should avoid.

The coffee can be 8 to 12 ounces regular coffee sweetened with sugar or stevia. If you have a habit of buying coffee at your favorite coffee house (e.g., Starbucks), please make sure you stick to regular coffee. Avoid the Frappuccinos and lattes, because they will add substantial amounts of calories to your diet.

In addition to boosting energy, coffee has many other health benefits, including lowering the risk of developing diabetes type 2, lowering body fat, and protecting the brain and liver. If you're not a coffee drinker, you may substitute the coffee with a cup of tea.

The coffee, together with the Greek yogurt will suppress hunger for a number of hours. You should not feel hungry for 3-4 hours (until lunch).

Lunch

For lunch, you're going to replace what you would usually eat for lunch three times per week with FAGE Greek yogurt. Use 12 to 16 ounces of FAGE Greek yogurt (depending on your weight and calorie requirements); it can be either 0% or 2% fat.

To flavor the yogurt, you can combine the yogurt with either fresh fruit or a jam/jelly. I have been using Bonne Mamman jelly to flavor my yogurt, as it mixes well with the yogurt, and adds a nice flavor.

This is going to be the hardest part of this plan, because most of you probably will not find it very appetizing to eat this much yogurt for lunch. Stick with it, and in a number of weeks, you will be rewarded with a better insulin response and weight loss. Here I recommend that you start slowly (begin with once a week and build up from there) in order for your digestive system to adjust. In case you're worried about being lactose intolerant, I have an entire chapter devoted to this topic (chapter 6).

The Greek yogurt will also fill you up. It adds bulk to your gut and adds good bacteria as well. If you didn't have an egg for breakfast, you can have an egg for lunch, in addition to the Greek yogurt. Do not worry about increasing cholesterol, because increasing your cholesterol by eating foods that are high in cholesterol (such as eggs) is a myth. Most of the cholesterol we eat will go straight through us. Our bodies produce most of the cholesterol that is needed for the body to function.

The main purpose of this change is that, three times a week, you replace your regular (*energy-dense*) lunch with Greek yogurt that is high in protein, is nutrient-dense and adds bulk and good bacteria to your gut.

Probiotic Drink

Kevita is a bubbly probiotic drink fermented with a water kefir culture, and comes in 10 different flavors. You may have seen many dairy kefir drinks, but water kefir cultures are different. With this probiotic drink, you add billions of good bacteria to your gut, which will aid your digestion and stimulate your immune system.

You'll add the Kevita probiotic drink two to three times per week to your diet (initially 3 times per week, tapering off to 2 times per week minimum after 3 months).

Make sure you'll buy the regular probiotic drink and not Kombucha. Kombucha is a fermented probiotic drink based on tea, and contains a different blend of bacteria. You may drink Kombucha later in the plan, but for now, stick to the regular Kevita probiotic drink.

The goal of the probiotic drink is to add good bacteria to your gut. Adding good bacteria will reduce all the unwanted issues that come with a less-than-healthy diet. It will reduce the bloating, it will reduce inflammation, decrease constipation as well as food cravings. Strangely enough, this also seems to be *brand-specific*. I've tried to drink other probiotic drinks, but none worked. I even tried probiotic powders and pills, but those didn't have the same effect as Kevita. For some reason, the probiotic blend in the Kevita drink will make sure that the good bacteria get properly taken up by your gut.

Cheese as a Snack

Feeling hungry in between meals? I recommend eating (Mini) Babybel cheese as a snack. Do this at least one to three times a day. You may pick the regular Babybel cheese or the cheddar Babybel cheese, but don't use the light version. There is something about the Babybel cheese in combination with the probiotic drink and the FAGE Greek yogurt that will jump-start your weight loss (you can read about why this is later in this chapter).

Drink Plenty of Water Throughout the Day

It's important to keep your body hydrated with water. Stay away from sodas and other drinks. You may feel hungry, when in fact, you could actually be thirsty.

Throughout the day, it's highly recommended that you drink a few glasses of regular water with a few drops of lemon juice. For lemon juice, use the Volcano Lemon Burst lemon juice. It's also brand-specific. I've used other brands of lemon juice, but other brands don't have the same effect, and don't taste as good. You may also use half a teaspoon of fresh lemon juice, but I find the concentrated lemon juice easier to use.

The goal of adding lemon juice to your water is to make your body more alkaline. Typical western diets are making our bodies become too acidic. Examples of foods that cause our body to become too acidic after digestion are sugar, alcohol, processed foods, trans-fats, pizza, white bread and meats.

Symptoms of acidification are fatigue, weight gain, depression, anxiety, dry skin, headaches, inflammation, candida overgrowth and ulcers.

Lemons, limes and concentrated lemon juice, despite being so acidic, can make you become **more alkaline**. This is mostly due to the mineral and electrolyte content of lemons and limes. Once the lemon juice has been metabolized, the minerals taken up by the blood (mostly potassium and sodium) will have an *alkalizing effect*.

For water, you can use filtered or spring water. Do not use tap water if the water company in your area adds fluoride to the drinking water, as fluoride can disrupt your metabolism. Drinking water throughout the day will keep you hydrated and also keep hunger at bay.

Dinner

For dinner, prepare a healthy dinner from scratch. And by *"from scratch,"* I mean fresh vegetables and fresh meat or protein - nothing frozen.

Make sure that you don't eat the same starch every day. So, pasta one day, potatoes the next, maybe some rice or quinoa or couscous.

Don't try to cut calories on your dinner. If your daily caloric intake is supposed to be 1800 calories, spent at least 30% on dinner. This will be at least 600 calories.

For cooking, only use healthy oils such as olive oil, avocado oil or coconut oil. It's a big misconception that you have to limit the amount of oil you use in cooking. Most of the time, the oil is used for frying or sautéing, therefore, most of the oil will remain in the pan after you take the food out. These oils are important for your brain's health.

You also want to make sure your dinner has a **high fat to carb ratio**. You don't want to limit your calories for dinner, otherwise, you will feel hungry right before going to bed; this hunger makes you indulge in late-night snacking, which is counterproductive.

You may ask yourself, *"Why does this work so well?"* or *"How can I trust that this will work for me?"*

The following chapter discusses the science behind this diet and why Greek yogurt, probiotics and cheese are so good for weight loss.

THE SCIENCE BEHIND THIS DIET

Probiotics and Weight Loss

Several studies have shown that there is a close relationship between your diet and the gut flora (the microorganisms living together in your gut, sometimes referred to as the **gut microbiome**): your diet determines the role and structure of the gut microbiome (the good and bad bacteria).

An imbalance in the gut microbiome can be caused by certain dietary and environmental factors (including consuming too many processed foods), which causes the overgrowth of bad bacteria.

In one particular study, researchers looked at mice and fed them either a high-fat diet or a high-carbohydrate diet. Both groups of mice showed increases in body weight during the first nine weeks.

However, as soon as they **added probiotics** to their diet during the last four weeks, both groups of mice **lost weight**.

The researchers further observed that a diet high in sugar had a more negative effect on the microbiome compared to a high-fat diet.

Another study looked at the differences in gut microbiome composition between lean college students and obese students. The study concluded that the microbiome in overweight college students was *less diverse* than in students who were considered lean.

Other studies have found a positive relationship between a diverse microbiome and digestion.

Several studies have found that probiotics are highly effective for improving BMI (Body Mass Index)* and body weight, and for increasing fat loss.

For example, in studies where they compared fat rats to lean rats, they discovered that the obese rats had increased fasting glucose levels, and increased insulin and insulin resistance, when compared to the lean rats.

Several studies in humans have made the same observation. They found that probiotics reduce BMI and total body fat, especially fat in the belly area. Also, they

46

found that people who took **probiotics** had **reduced insulin levels** and **reduced insulin resistance**.

The Effect Of Probiotics On Hormones Regulating Appetite

In another recent study, researchers studied the effect of probiotics on the levels of certain hormones produced in the gut, and their effect on body weight and obesity.

The main hormone that they studied was *ghrelin*, which is a hunger hormone. Ghrelin, which is produced in the gut, promotes hunger (and food intake), and increases fat deposits. If ghrelin levels stay too high for a long period, insulin resistance can occur.

Researchers found that the consumption of probiotics through yogurt for example, lowered the levels of the ghrelin hormone, and *promoted the generation of heat and lowered obesity*.

Another hormone that was studied was the hormone **leptin**. Leptin (from the Greek word *'lepton'*, meaning 'thin' or 'light) is a protein hormone predominantly made by fat cells. Its primary role is to regulate energy balance. Leptin has a major effect on appetite and feeding behavior.

A particular probiotic bacterium, *L. plantarum* is able to suppress the leptin hormone, and consequently, reduce the cell size of fat tissue cells.

The Effect Of Greek Yogurt On Muscle

In yet another study, researchers looked at the effect of Greek yogurt on muscle composition. The study involved two groups of college-aged students. One group was the Greek yogurt group, and the other group was the pudding group.

The students were asked to eat a yogurt or a pudding right after a workout, however, the groups didn't know what they were receiving because the Greek yogurt and the (placebo) pudding were made to taste the same.

Researchers also make sure that the two groups received the same amount of calories each day. The two groups each consumed either the yogurt or the pudding right after a weight lifting workout session.

The consumption of Greek yogurt during a 12-week exercise program resulted in more strength, more muscle thickness and better body composition in the students who ate it than the students in the carbohydrate (pudding) control group.

Because yogurt has a high protein content and is able to increase lean muscle mass and ***lower fat deposits***, yogurt should be considered a valuable health food source.

Effect of *Prebiotics* on Weight and Appetite Hormones

Other studies looked at the effect of *prebiotics* on weight and appetite. **Prebiotics** are the undigested material in foods (such as fiber) that are used by the microbiome bacteria.

Examples of prebiotics are inulin (a type of indigestible fiber present in some yogurts, onion, leeks and asparagus), galacto-oligosaccharides (GOS) and fructose oligo-saccharides (FOS)[1].

The addition of these prebiotics to your diet result in an increase of certain good bacteria of the microbiome, reduction of the hunger hormone Ghrelin and a reduction in overall food intake.

Inulin is present in dandelion greens, bananas, certain yogurts, onions, leeks and asparagus. FOS can be found in onions and burdock root. GOS can be found in legumes, cashews, hummus, soy and milk.

The Magic Of MCTs (Medium Chain Triglycerides)

Medium-chain triglycerides (MCTs) are a type of fat found in oils such as coconut oil palm kernel oil and are also present in dairy such as butter and **yogurt**. Recently, MCTs have gained attention due to the fact that they are linked to increased energy and appetite control. So what exactly are MCTs and what are the potential health benefits?

The types of MCTs

MCTs are a type of saturated fat with medium chain fatty acids, which contain between 6 and 12 carbon atoms. When the body uses fat as an energy source, MCTs are the preferred source. This is mostly because medium-chain triglycerides are easily absorbed by the liver and are used for energy quicker to provide fuel for the body.

The few types of MCTs are the following:

- Caproic acid (C6)
- Caprylic acid (C8)
- Capric acid (C10)
- Lauric acid (C12)

Caprylic Acid (C8) and Capric Acid (C10) can be found in the milk of some mammals, while Lauric acid (C12) is the main fatty acid found in coconut oil and palm kernel oil.

Grass-fed butter contains approximately 8% MCTs and **full-fat yogurt contains about 8-9% of MCTs.**

Health Benefits Of MCTs

MCTs have many health benefits, including weight loss, increased energy and improved gut health.

MCT oil seems to help with weight loss by promoting the feeling of being full. When MCT oils are present in your meal (whether it's breakfast, lunch or dinner), you will feel fuller longer which helps to prevent you from over eating. MCTs also have been reported to increase thermogenesis, a metabolic process in which your body burns calories to produce heat. This in turn, can also result in weight loss.

MCTs are a quick source of energy and can enter cells easily. MCTs are converted into ketones in the liver, which provides a more efficient source of energy for the brain resulting in increased focus and concentration.

While MCTs are a type of saturated fat, they are considered heart-healthy. Many research studies have suggested that MCTs offer protective effects on cardiovascular health by improving serum lipid profiles. A number of studies have also demonstrated that MCT supplementation has a positive effect on cognition, both in healthy individuals and in people suffering from Alzheimer's disease and other neurological conditions.

MCT oil has become popular as a dietary supplement. It is similar in appearance as olive oil and can be added to hot beverages such as coffee and tea. Most people can tolerate up to 6 tablespoons of MCTs per day (taken throughout the day), but it is generally recommended to start slowly (for example one teaspoon per day) in order to give the gut time to adjust to the increased levels of fat. Signs of over-supplementation of MCTs are loose stools, diarrhea, bloating and cramping.

MCTs are antibacterial and anti-fungal. They help to control bacterial and fungal overgrowth in the gut, helping to *restore microbiome balance*.

While MCT supplements can be beneficial to your health, consuming yogurt and cooking with butter are two natural ways to strengthen your gut's microbiome and will help you reach your weight loss goals.

How Hormones Like GLP-1 Help With Weight Loss

Your gut produces a certain hormone called **GLP-1** (Glucagon-like peptide-1), which regulates the amount of sugar in your blood through the pancreas. It also tells your body that you have had enough to eat and slows down the movement along your intestines to allow your food to be digested. This system is sometimes referred to as the *"colonic brake"*.

A **healthy microbiome** (the good bacteria in your gut) takes components of the food you eat that cannot be digested - such as fiber and polyphenols (the compounds that give vegetables its color for example) - and transforms them into molecules that stimulate hormones such as **GLP-1** to control your appetite and metabolism.

That is why a healthy gut and a properly functioning microbiome are so important for regulating food cravings and metabolism. Earlier in this book I talked about the importance of eliminating processed foods as much as possible. Food processing, which was invented to enhance taste and improve shelf life, removes bioactive molecules such as fiber and polyphenols that help to regulate this system.

A diet with a reduced intake of these bioactive compounds will result in a less diverse microbiome and could ultimately result in weight gain, elevated blood sugars and insulin insensitivity.

How GLP-1 agonist drugs work

During the last few years, appetite modulating GLP-1 drugs such as semaglutide have become extremely popular. These class of drugs mimic GLP-1 and trick the body that you're full, thereby helping people eat less and lose weight.

These drugs were initially developed to control blood sugar and were very helpful to patients with Type 2 diabetes. These drugs have become very successful in helping control blood sugar and have assisted individuals in losing 15% of their weight over 12 months on average.

These drugs are broken down very slowly and that's the reason that patients only have to be injected once a week or twice a month. These drugs target the GLP-1 receptors in the brain where they lower your appetite in a powerful way. Since they target the brain, they also curb other behaviors such as drinking, smoking, compulsive shopping and other addictive behaviors.

Should people who only need to lose a little weight be on these medications?

These drugs are not without side effects. Since they stay in your system for such a long time, they also trigger side effects such as nausea, vomiting, diarrhea and constipation. More severe side effects include inflammation of the pancreas and paralysis of the stomach. These drugs also seem to induce loss of lean muscle mass, in particular in the absence of exercise, and can sometimes be visible in the faces of people taking these drugs.

Despite the many side effects and hefty price tag, many people are tempted to take these medications, hoping for a quick fix for their weight loss goals. But how to safely get off these medications and return to a regular lifestyle *without significant weight gain*, proves problematic. It is also not known what the long-term effects of these drugs are.

Peptides that Control Your Appetite

Think of peptides as small chunks of protein. Several peptides that are important for appetite control and lipid (fat) metabolism are produced in the gut. These peptides have also been found in cow's milk whey and cheese whey. This suggests that peptides found in milk and cheese may be important for a healthy human diet because of their biological and physiological properties.

As you have seen from the evidence presented above, probiotics, prebiotics and peptides present in yogurt, cheese and the probiotic drink all contribute to a **lowered appetite, increased lean muscle mass and increased fat burning**.

Re-building your gut's microbiome by following the diet discussed in this book in combination with more whole foods, may be the best way to control appetite, increase metabolism, lose weight and avoid the need for these types of medications.

IN SUMMARY, during the next phase, you're going to replace your breakfast and your lunch with Greek yogurt, you're going to add the Kevita probiotic drink two to three times per week, and you're going to snack on Babybel cheese.

During the next two to three months, you will experience less food cravings and increased energy. This can ultimately reverse insulin resistance in the long run, and as a result, you will start to lose weight in problem areas such as the stomach area, the hips and thighs.

6

WHAT IF YOU CANNOT HAVE DAIRY?

At this point, you may be wondering *"Why so much dairy? I won't be able to eat dairy as I'm lactose intolerant."*

This chapter will address these concerns, discuss the levels of lactose present in Greek yogurt and cheese and offer some excellent **dairy alternatives** based on cashews and coconut milk.

It is estimated that 65% of all people have some form of *lactose intolerance*, a condition where there is not enough of the enzyme lactase present in the gut to break down the complex sugar lactose that is found in dairy.

Lactase breaks down lactose into glucose and galactose. Lactose that isn't broken down can cause bloating, cramps and diarrhea in people who are lactose intolerant. However, most people do not have to eliminate all dairy from their diet unless they're severely lactose intolerant (meaning their body does not produce *any* lactase).

For most people with milder cases, a small cup size of Greek yogurt (as is described in **Chapter 4** for breakfast) and a small piece of cheese as a snack won't trigger digestive issues due to their lower lactose content.

If you're worried about consuming dairy, you can start with small amounts and gradually increase or switch to dairy alternatives such as coconut or cashew yogurts.

How much lactose is present in Greek yogurt?

Greek yogurt is different from other yogurts in how it is produced. Greek yogurt is a *strained* yogurt, which means that the whey (a milk protein) is taken out of the yogurt. When the whey is removed, a large part of the lactose is removed as well.

Greek yogurt contains about half as much lactose as regular yogurts. The significant reduction in lactose in Greek yogurt also attributes to its tart taste.

Greek yogurts also have *"live active cultures"* (*aka* probiotics or the good bacteria), which will help to digest any leftover lactose when the yogurt hits your gut. These good bacteria are important as they feed on the lactose (for example *Lactobacillus bulgaricus, Lactobacillus acidophilus, Lactobacillus casei*) and eat up much of the lactose that is left in the yogurt.

The many probiotics present in Greek yogurt are beneficial to digestion, gut health and your immunity. Furthermore, yogurt contains essential nutrients such as protein, calcium, potassium, phosphorus, vitamin B-12 among others. The fact that Greek yogurt is low in calories and high in protein, makes it the perfect food for anyone who wants to lose weight.

Yogurt alternatives

If you're still worried about consuming dairy and would like to know about a good alternative, coconut yogurt and yogurt made from cashews are good choices.

Coconut yogurt will have the same micro-nutrients as regular yogurt such as calcium and vitamin B-12, but it won't have the same amount of protein as regular yogurt. However, coconuts contain high amounts of *medium-chain fatty triglycerides* (**MCTs**) that have been linked to weight loss and reduced incidences of Alzheimer's disease. I discussed MCTs in the previous chapter.

Another good yogurt alternative is **Forager Project** Cashew yogurt. It is made from cashew milk and coconut cream and contains a good amount of probiotics (*S. Thermophilus, L. Plantarum, L. Acidophilus, Bifidus, L. Lactis*). Forager's Cashew yogurt is higher in protein than coconut yogurt. **Forager Project** yogurts are organic, gluten-free, dairy-free and free of fillers and thickeners.

Lactose Content Of Cheese

As long as you eat aged cheeses (think Parmesan, Cheddar or Swiss) that have been aged 6 months or more, lactose should not prove an issue as those cheeses contain almost no lactose. The enzymes that are used to make these cheeses, over time break down all the lactose present, so after 6 months time there won't be any lactose left.

What is the **lactose content of Babybel cheese** I introduced in chapter 4? According to the manufacturer, Babybel cheese does not contain any lactose, as all lactose is being eliminated during the draining and fermentation process, making Babybel cheese a perfect snack for lactose intolerant individuals.

SECTION III

**Making It All
Work**

7

YOU MAY HAVE QUESTIONS
IMPORTANT THINGS TO KNOW FOR OPTIMAL RESULTS

I f you have followed this plan for a few months now, you're well on your way to permanent weight loss, and you'll start to see results. You may notice increased energy, reduced food cravings, and that your skin and hair look healthier.

Don't worry if you're not losing as much weight as you thought you would, because it will take a long time before your metabolism catches up. How long or short this journey is for you is mostly dependent on how much non-organic foods and processed foods you were eating before and how many sodas and fast foods you have eliminated from your diet.

Just remember that you didn't gain all the weight in a few weeks; it took years for you to become overweight.

So, it is reasonable to expect that it will take as long or maybe longer to lose the weight. I implore you, please don't lose hope. Even little steps will get you there. The most important thing is to stick with the plan and to implement some of the changes every day. Even the smallest changes can lead to big results. By now, you should be familiar with the main steps of this plan.

However, there might be some information that you're not totally aware of, and this is what this chapter is all about. It will address some of the questions you may have, and will also provide additional information that will make this plan even better.

The topics I'm covering in this chapter range from how to deal with restaurant or takeout food, and how to deal with stress, to how long it will take to see results. So, please read on, and read every question because the information is really important for the entire plan to work.

Question 1: I have been following this plan for two months now. When will I see any results?

To see any results with this plan, you will have to take into consideration that it's dependent on many factors, such as your rate of metabolism, your age, your food intake, the type of food you're eating every day, your activity level and how long you've been following this plan.

On average, I would say that after two months, you will start to see changes in body composition, and reduced food cravings. You will also feel better overall.

You have to remember that the primary focus of your brain is survival. With this survival mechanism in place, any changes in calories will be met with resistance. For example, if you start to eat less calories every day and you implement all the changes that I've talked about in the previous chapters, it will take about two months before your metabolism is changed enough for you to see any changes in weight, body fat composition and feelings of hunger. But rest assured that once you're in the *"zone,"* you will actually see changes every day. These changes will appear as weight loss, less hunger throughout today, better skin and better health.

Question 2: How long do I need to stay on this diet?

This question came up after I published the first edition of this book. Remember that the *long-term goal* of this plan is to have a healthy gut with a healthy microbiome, a healthier diet with less food cravings and to achieve your weight loss goals. Based on the science behind this diet plan, you know that sustaining a healthy microbiome is important for reaching these long term goals. The Greek yogurt and probiotic drink are the main contributors to this healthier microbiome. That is not to say that you will need to consume that much yogurt or drink as much probiotic drink forever.

Once you have reached your weight loss goals and you feel better, I would suggest that you slowly taper off the yogurt and probiotic drink (*but not completely*) and see how your body reacts in terms of food cravings and weight gain. How slow you do this is dependent on your body and personal circumstances, but you could start tapering off by consuming 10% less yogurt and probiotic drink for 3-4 weeks and see how your body reacts. The idea here is that you want to keep your gut and microbiome in top shape so that you won't re-gain any weight. This means you'll have to consume a certain amount of prebiotics and probiotics each week to keep the microbiome in balance. How much you'll need to consume (in terms of Greek yogurt, the probiotic drink and prebiotics coming from certain vegetables), is person dependent. That is why you should taper off slowly and see how your body responds.

Question 3: How do you deal with restaurant or takeout food?

Of course, you can go out to restaurants and have takeout food every now or then, because it will be unnatural not to do so. Plus, it is never a good idea to feel guilty about your food choices.

The focus here should be *"What are the long term goals of your diet strategy?"* If you do decide to go out to eat in a restaurant or to take out food from a restaurant, it's always better to go to a restaurant that uses fresh ingredients and prepares the food from scratch.

However, this might be easier said than done. As you can witness in the TV series '*Kitchen Nightmares*' by chef Gordon Ramsay, there are many restaurants that cut corners by using frozen foods, foods that come out of bags, foods that are heated in a microwave, and by deep-frying your food. A giant red flag for a bad restaurant is using a multi-page menu with items that are not in season and people leaving with too many doggie bags.

While it's best to avoid restaurants that use processed foods, sometimes it may not be possible. Occasionally eating at a bad restaurant will not derail your weight loss goals in the long run. As long as the overall trend of your diet is mostly whole foods (fresh ingredients with plenty of pre- and probiotics) and you keep processed foods to a minimum, you should be fine.

Question 4: How does alcohol fit in with this plan?

With this plan, it's okay to consume alcohol a few times a week as long as you count the calories and add them to your daily calorie intake. If you know how many calories you consume each day (see chapter 3), you'll know how much you can consume and still stay on track with your weight loss goals.

Wine would be better than beer and also has the added benefit of containing a lot of antioxidants that are good for the overall health. Please note that red wine is slightly better than white wine with respect to weight loss. After you drink wine, do not forget to drink a glass of water with lemon juice before going to bed to hydrate your body and to counteract the acidity of the wine (see section about drinking water in Chapter 4).

If you prefer beer, I would suggest you limit beer to perhaps twice a month. The problem with beer is that it contains a lot of gluten. If you drink a lot of beer, the gluten will clash with your weight loss plan. Beer is also very dehydrating, and has a negative effect on the gut microbiome. Wine is a much better choice as it has a positive effect on the gut microbiome. However, I would suggest to limit wine to about twice a week as too much wine can disrupt your hormonal balance.

QUESTION 5: I love pizza. Can I still eat pizza?

Of course, you can still eat pizza, but remember that pizza is an *energy-dense food*. Before I get into recommendations as to the kinds of pizza you should consider, I need to explain what **enriched flour** is all about. Most pizzas (as do other baked goods) use enriched flour.

White flour has been used for ages. A few centuries ago, it was thought that dark flour was not as good as white flour. White flour was also considered a status symbol, as it was much more expensive than darker flour. Because of the chemical processing used to produce white flour, in the 1920s, factories came up with a process to add essential nutrients to the flour; hence, enriched flour was born.

Enriched flour was adopted in the 1940s as a means to improve the health of wartime soldiers both in Britain and the United States, while food was being rationed.

In order to produce flour, several grains have to be processed. During the first steps of flour processing, the bran and the germ of the seeds are removed, in order to improve shelf life.

During the later stages of flour processing, a chemical bleaching process is used to give the flour its white color. This bleaching process destroys many of the original nutrients that are present in flour. Enriching the flour ensures that these important nutrients are restored, and improve the quality of the flour. However, enriched flour is produced with so many chemicals, that it is not really healthy for you.

When you eat a lot of carbohydrate meals that are produced with enriched flour, you also absorb a lot of these chemicals used in the processing of that flour.

This will result in a lower metabolism in the long run, and inevitably, you'll start to gain weight.

In addition, the highly processed enriched flour will be absorbed by your body much faster than raw flour, and it will give you much higher sugar spikes. This excess sugar in the bloodstream will have to be processed by the liver, which will store some of it as fat.

You'll be surprised how many food products contain enriched flour; even organic food stores sell many breads and crackers that are made with enriched flour.

So, what kind of pizza can you eat with this plan; one that's healthy enough, and won't interfere with your metabolism? I would suggest that you take a look at *Oath Pizza* and *Jules Thin Crust Pizza*. Both pizza places produce a thin crust pizza that uses non-GMO, non-bromated and non-bleached flour.

Oath Pizza's crust is made with 100% pure grain North Dakota Mills flour that is flash seared in pure olive oil. The crust is then grilled in a convection oven for just ninety seconds, resulting in a tasty, buttery crust. Jules Thin Crust pizza uses high-gluten flour from Dakota Prairie, made from organic hard red spring wheat. Both pizza places use various organic toppings.

You may not be able to find these pizza places in your area; if that's the case, I would suggest that you look at similar pizza restaurants by comparing ingredients. Be sure to always pay especially close attention to the flour they use.

Question 6: How much and what kind of bread can I eat?

With this plan, I recommend that you limit your bread consumption to no more than 3-4 times a week, and preferably not on days that you have Greek yogurt for lunch (*low gluten days*).

Whole grain breads are better than white bread. When buying your bread, make sure that it is made with real, unbleached and unbromated flour, and not **enriched flour** (see previous question). This means that you'll have to read a few labels, but that is better than messing up your weight-loss efforts by unknowingly buying bread that is made with enriched flour.

Wholefoods sells many breads that are made with real flour, even the popular bake-at-home breads. Another good bread to buy is *Dave's Killer Bread*, which also comes as thin sliced bread and is made with real flour. Dave's Killer Bread is also available at regular grocery stores.

Question 7: How much red meat can I eat?

In general, red meat is more unhealthy than white meat. While I would suggest you limit red meat as much as possible, it is important to realize that red meat comes with so many qualities. Red meat bought in non-organic food stores is raised with a lot of hormones, produced with tons of chemicals and is simply not healthy.

If possible, buy only grass-fed organic beef. However, it is important to know that the high fat content of red meat is also not good for your heart. In addition, frequent consumption of red meat can make conditions such as hemorrhoids much, much worse.

Question 8: I don't eat dairy. Can I still benefit benefit from this plan?

I realize that this plan recommends the use of a lot of dairy in the form of Greek yogurt. Some people don't eat dairy because they don't like it, while there are others who don't eat dairy because they're sensitive to lactose.

If you're lactose intolerant, there exist plenty of dairy alternatives such as yogurt produced with cashews (see also Chapter 6).

Forager is a brand of dairy-free products that uses cashews to produce delicious milk and yogurt. Their products also contain various strains of good probiotics such as the strain *L. plantarum*. *L. plantarum* has been shown to suppress the leptin hormone, thereby reducing the size of fat deposits in the body.

Question 9: Do you have any recommendations for vegetarians?

Vegetarians can still benefit from this plan. The only suggestion I have is that you make sure that you eat enough protein every day. During the day, you will get enough protein from the Greek yogurt, but for dinner, make sure that you still eat enough protein. Some of this protein can come from tofu, seitan, beans or other vegetarian protein sources.

There are several good brands of organic plant-based meats that are high in protein. For example, Gardein makes several tasty plant-based 'Chicken' products made from seitan. Beyond Meat makes really good meat alternatives based on pea protein. Make sure you get your protein from a variety of sources, and not just from eggs. Do not eat eggs every day. As a vegetarian, you should also make sure you get enough vitamin B-12 and iron.

Question 10: Can I also eat nuts as a snack?

Yes, of course. Nuts are a perfect snack to eat in between meals. One of the best nuts to have as a snack is walnuts. **Walnuts can actually lower hunger cravings.** Peanuts are also good because they result in a *low insulin response.* The third nut that you could eat as a snack is cashew. Cashew is really good for you, as it is high in minerals, magnesium, copper and manganese. It is also good for the heart as it lowers cholesterol.

Walnuts, peanuts and cashews are great as a healthy snack, and can *boost your fat burning metabolism*. Try not to eat more than a small handful of nuts each time. Some nuts can be purchased in convenient 100 calorie packs. I would not recommend pistachios as a snack. They contain a lot of protein, but they are quite energy-dense, and they make you gain weight fairly fast.

Question 11: Would it help if I use apple cider vinegar?

Apple cider vinegar has become fairly popular in recent years, and is sometimes used together with a keto diet. Of course, you can use apple cider vinegar every day with this plan. I have tried it myself, but I find it a little bit hard to swallow because of the taste. But if you don't mind the taste, go ahead and use apple cider vinegar every day. It may actually help with increasing your weight loss.

Question 12: Isn't this plan almost like a keto diet?

There are some similarities with this plan and the keto diet. However, with a keto diet, you restrict carbohydrates so much, in order for the body to stay in ketosis. In ketosis, the body starts to burn fat instead of carbohydrates as an energy source. This is how a typical keto diet works; it limits your carbohydrates sources so that you stay in ketosis in order to burn fat. The keto diet has been reported to help people who suffer from seizures and epilepsy (see the movie "Fat: A documentary").

Although the keto diet has helped many people lose weight, I think that the keto diet has too many restrictions, which will not work in the long run. One reason is that the high fat content of the keto diet may not be healthy for longer periods. If you want to keep the weight off, the plan I have described in this book ensures that the insulin response stays low and stable throughout the day until dinner time.

Question 13: Does stress make me overweight?

Stress is a major contributor to weight gain. The hormone cortisol, which is released by elevated stress levels, promotes weight gain. In order to reduce stress, you can perform breathing exercises a few times a day. Take a moment to splash your face with cool water in the morning or at night. This releases chemicals in the brain that will reduce stress. It is almost like jumping into a pool or ocean.

In order to reduce stress even more, it's important not to have your cell phone next to your bed at night, not to read emails an hour before going to bed and to allow at least eight hours of restful sleep. If you have trouble falling asleep, you may benefit from taking melatonin.

Reduced melatonin levels are linked to increased weight gain and fat deposits.

Question 14: I have trouble sleeping. Is a lack of sleep causing my weight issues?

Yes, see also previous question. If you have trouble sleeping, you may have lower levels of melatonin. Lack of sleep and lower levels of melatonin have been linked to an increase in body weight and increased fat deposits. It is therefore important that you get a full night (eight hours) of restful sleep without interruptions or distractions. If you have chronic lack of sleep, it is important to take some melatonin in order to get a restful night of sleep.

Question 15: I'm worried about what others may say about me when I eat yogurt for lunch?

What you eat for lunch is your business. Never worry what others may say about your food choices. This is your health, and you should never give in to peer pressure. If it helps, you could eat the FAGE Greek yogurt for lunch on the weekends, and then just one more time during the week. But promise yourself never to give in to peer pressure and skip your plan in order to join your colleagues with what they're eating for lunch. Most companies' cafeterias sell food that is overly processed, and often, fried.

Question 16: Should I buy food in bulk?

Buying food in bulk is never a good idea. Most healthy foods don't come in bulk anyway. The food they sell in so-called membership clubs are heavily processed with tons of chemicals and can make you fat. Plus, if you buy more than a few days' worth of food, you run into the problem of not having enough storage space in your fridge. When you have that much food in your fridge, you start to use excuses like "I/*we really should finish this before it expires.*" Because you feel guilty about throwing food away, you start to eat more than you should. This is counterproductive and will not be helpful for your long-term weight loss efforts.

Question 17: Are there any other apps that are useful for losing weight?

I have found that another app called "*My Fitness Pal*" does a good job in giving you insights to how **energy-dense** certain foods are. Take a look at a particular food you've just had and enter it into My Fitness Pal. For example, enter a steak, a burger or a pizza. It will tell you exactly how many minutes you have to exercise or walk to burn off the calories. Of course, this is just for illustrative and entertainment purposes. It will give you a good idea of how **energy-dense** certain foods are.

Question 18: What sweetener should I use in my coffee or tea?

I would stick with natural sweeteners. You want to stay away from man-made chemicals, also known as unnatural sweeteners, such as aspartame and sucralose. Man-made sweeteners will trick the brain, interfere with the insulin response and eventually lower your metabolism.

For the most part, stick with sugar. If you would like to limit your sugar consumption, you can replace half of it with **Stevia** extract. Stevia extract is great because it's very sweet and stimulates weight loss at the same time.

If you decide to use Stevia as a sweetener, I would recommend that you buy a Stevia product without erythritol. Often, stevia is packaged with erythritol to increase the sweetness.

Erythritol is an alcohol-type sugar that is present in low amounts in fruits and vegetables and is also generated inside our own cells as part of our normal metabolism. However, when used as a sweetener, erythritol levels are usually 1,000 times higher than found in natural foods.

Recently, erythritol and related sweeteners have been linked to a high risk of cardiovascular events (such as heart attack and stroke). In one study, blood erythritol levels increased 1,000-fold after drinking a beverage sweetened with erythritol. Erythritol levels stayed high for several days and resulted in an increase in blood clot formation. More research is needed, but for now I would suggest only using pure Stevia.

Another popular natural sweetener is **agave syrup**. I would not recommend the use of agave syrup as a sweetener, because it contains a lot of fructose.

Question 19: What is the best time to weigh myself?

The best time to weigh yourself is in the morning, right before taking a shower and after you've had your breakfast. Whatever time you choose to weigh yourself, make sure you keep the time consistent. Step on the scale without clothes. Don't become obsessed with your weight, as everyone's weight will fluctuate from day to day. Your weight is dependent on a number of factors, such as how much exercise you did the day before, the kind of food you had the day before (not just the calories), your hormones and your mood.

Don't blame yourself if your weight increases one day. Weight fluctuations are normal, and if you're trying to lose weight, just pay attention to the weekly trend. You want to prevent any feelings of guilt. If you have been following this plan for a while, and then you have been to a party or notice you have gained weight during the holidays, just remember that the weight will come off fairly easy (usually within a few days).

Question 20: I'm still having incredible food cravings. What can I do?

You may still have persistent food cravings, even after you have been implementing this plan. There could be several reasons.

First, make sure you eat the correct number of calories each day. One of the reasons that you still have food cravings (mostly sugar or carbohydrate cravings) is Candida (yeast) overgrowth. Many people suffer from Candida overgrowth in the gut. Candida can cause bloating, gas, constipation, fatigue, low energy and low metabolism. In order to get rid of Candida, you could consider a so-called Candida cleanse. Look up 'Candida cleanse near me' on Google to find healthcare professionals in your area who can help you get rid of Candida safely.

The second reason you are still having food cravings, is that you may be eating snacks between meals that contain hidden sugars. These kind of snacks are considered processed foods and manufacturers often add sugars to make the food taste better. These sugars can be found on the label under "added sugars". Your brain wants to hold on to the sugar high and when the sugar level in the blood drops quickly, you will experience these bad food cravings. Take a look at what you're eating and if the food or snacks contain a lot of added sugars, try to replace it with something else.

Question 21: Are there any other things that can help with weight loss?

There are a few additional things you can consider. One is to eat blueberries regularly. Blueberries are high in antioxidants and are anti-inflammatory. They can also improve insulin sensitivity and contain prebiotics that will help with your gut health.

Health supplements you should consider are Stinging Nettle Root extract and L-Carnitine. Stinging Nettle Root extract is great for lowering the estrogen-like effects of certain foods such as tofu, avocados and wine, while L-Carnitine boosts cellular energy and helps mobilize fatty acids. L-Carnithine can certainly help with weight loss, especially when taken after a workout session.

8

SHOULD YOU EXERCISE?

EXERCISE TO BOOST YOUR METABOLISM

When you use this plan, there is no need to exercise in order to lose weight. You will lose weight simply by following the steps I have described in this book. However, adding exercise to your daily routine will help you lose weight even faster, as exercise will boost your metabolism and will also increase your muscle strength. Exercise will make you healthier in the long run.

It doesn't have to be very complicated to add exercise to your daily routine. You can start by adding 10 to 20 minutes of walking every day. And you don't need to invest in expensive exercise equipment either.

An excuse that many people use is that they don't have time to exercise, but that's just a misconception.

There's plenty of time each day, and you can definitely find 10 to 20 minutes to set aside for some exercise.

WALKING

Walking is about the easiest exercise you can add to your daily routine. You can walk around the block, walk through your neighborhood or walk in the park.

Some people have recently called walking the most *underrated form of exercise*. Walking for at least 20 minutes a day can reduce your risk for heart disease by 30%. It can also relieve stress and anxiety, and boost your mood. Studies have shown that walking can lower your risk for dementia and Alzheimer's disease.

The average American walks about **5,000 steps** a day. That is a little over 2 miles a day. These steps can be from walking back and forth at the office, doing chores around the house or by intentionally going for a walk. While walking 10,000 steps a day used to be a healthy goal, new studies have found that anywhere between 4,000 and 7,000 steps may be enough to see health benefits. The health app on the iPhone is a great way to see how active you are on any given day and will give you great insights on your walking trends.

Most people don't even think about how much they walk each day. It really isn't that hard to increase the amount you're walking by a little. If you have a dog, then of course, you're forced to walk every day. But even if you don't have a dog, you can add walking to your daily routine, by setting aside some time after work or before work. Even walking during your lunch break can help.

Did you know that by walking 10 minutes, you can burn 100 calories? This may not sound like much, but if you do this every day, it will add up. It will help you burn more calories every day and lose the weight even faster. Plus, it's good for your bones, your muscles and your heart.

WEIGHTLIFTING

Lifting weights is another form of exercise that's easy to incorporate in your daily routine. It increases muscle strength, and will result in increased lean muscle mass. Lifting weights is good for your heart and your circulation, and will help you lose extra calories.

Each pound of muscle burns between 30 and 60 calories each day in resting state. That is a heck of a lot more than what fat tissue burns each day (0 cal).

You don't have to invest in expensive weightlifting equipment. You also don't have to spend a lot of money on gym memberships. The problem with gym memberships is that people usually join a gym in January right after the new year. They spent a lot of money on a gym membership and then forget about it a few months later and never make it to the gym again. That is a complete waste of money and time.

The best way to do weightlifting at home is to buy free weights or dumbbells. You could buy five-pound, ten-pound or twenty-pound dumbbells, which cost about $25 to $150 for each pair, depending on their weight. These dumbbells fit easily underneath a bed or a desk, and all you have to do is spend 10 to 20 minutes, two to three times a week, lifting weights.

There are many different exercises you can do with free weights. Examples of exercises you can do at home with free weights are bicep curls, upright row, squat to overhead press, dumbbell punch, dumbbell delt raise and more. Just do a quick Google search on exercises with free weights, and you'll get plenty of examples and videos.

Before you start lifting weights, make sure your body is properly warmed up by doing some squats for two minutes. This is to prevent any injury. Do each weightlifting exercise for 10 to 15 reps, and rest 10 to 20 seconds in between exercises. Do at least one round of exercises and mix them up with stomach crunches.

Many people join gyms in order to work out. But going to the gym can be tough. Gyms are often overcrowded, while machines that you would like to use are either occupied or broken. It's also difficult to go to the gym by yourself as it is much easier to skip when you're feeling unmotivated or if something unexpected comes up. For those reasons, it is much better to join a gym with a friend, colleague from work or family member and meet at the gym at a specific time each week. That way you stay motivated and are accountable for each other's progress.

Another benefit of strength training is that you will burn calories long after the workout is over (*afterburn effect*). You will get the most benefit from working out when you combine some form of aerobic exercise with weight training. For example, 10-20 minutes on a treadmill, and 30-40 minutes of fairly intense weight training will give you the most benefits in terms of increasing lean muscle mass, increasing metabolism and burning fat.

PERSONAL TRAINER

When you work out by yourself in a gym, it's easy to become lazy or do less than what you're capable of, and be easily distracted. If you can afford it, I would highly recommend working with a personal trainer.

If you work with a personal trainer, you're less likely to cancel the workout sessions because you will lose money. Some personal trainers work with couples, so, if you have a partner or a friend who would like to join you, with some personal trainers, you can do that. The workout will be more fun, and it will also help you keep each other motivated.

Working with a personal trainer is beneficial because the workout is completely tailored to you, and the exercises are chosen based on your level of strength. Because of this level of personalized fitness, you will prevent injuries, while your workout is optimized to maximize your results.

A high-intensity workout is not only good to lift your mood and reduce stress, but you feel energized and motivated. A personal training program will improve your core strength, build lean muscle and increase your metabolism.

When I first started working with a personal trainer, I was amazed at how out of shape I was. I considered myself relatively healthy, but the first couple of months working out were really tough. I often felt totally out of breath and felt really nauseous at the end of each workout, but I stuck with it, and now, I feel better than ever.

BIKING

Biking is a great form of exercise. It builds muscle strength, and is great for the circulation and the heart. However, not everybody can bike easily in their neighborhood or town. That's where Peloton comes in. Peloton is a stationary bike workout system that came to the market in 2012. The system consists of a stationary bike, with a screen in which you can follow On-Demand classes. The bike itself is fairly expensive, so if you're not sure you want to invest in such an expensive piece of equipment, you could ask around your local gyms and find out if there's a local gym that has some of these bikes available. Or perhaps if a friend has a bike you can try out.

If you have seen the Peloton ads on TV, you'll know the kind of image they try to portray. Based on my own experience with Peloton, I can tell you that whatever they portray in their ads isn't similar to the people that I see on the Facebook Peloton groups at all. Most people who work out on Peloton are just regular people who want to become healthier, lose some weight and have fun doing it. If you're not completely sure about Peloton, I recommend that you try out a bike from a friend or at a gym, and give it a try.

Of all the possible exercises, Peloton is the only exercise that can really jump-start your weight loss. They have classes ranging from 10 to 60 minutes in length, with all kinds of instructors. For example, you can easily start out with a 10-minute class, then go to a 20-minute class and build up to a 45-minute class. With a 45-minute class, you can easily burn up to 700 calories.

From my own experience, I can tell you that it took about four weeks before I saw some weight loss from Peloton, despite that I was burning close to 700 calories five days a week; it clearly shows you that the body is really resistant to weight loss, and it will take a long time before you start to see any results. Of course, it's not all about the weight loss; it's also about becoming healthier and having a good time. Doing such intense workout will make you release a lot of endorphins.

The longer workout sessions on the Peloton are also excellent for circulation and for heart health. It is always a good idea to do a 10-minute cool-down exercise after you spend 45 minutes on the bike.

While it is possible to work out on the Peloton every day, I would suggest 24-48 hour rests between workouts, especially if you have done a high-intensity workout, longer than 30 minutes. If you over-train, you'll run the risk that you damage muscle tissue. Losing muscle tissue has a negative effect on your metabolism.

Adding exercise to your routine can be really beneficial to your health, and will make you burn extra calories.

Frequent exercise is good for your mood, circulation and bones. It also makes you feel younger. Any form of exercise will help, and if you add exercise to your daily routine in small steps, you'll be more likely to stick with it.

9

NEXT STEPS

In this book, I have covered the many reasons why most diets don't work, and why you're not losing weight. The information I've given you is backed by scientific facts. If you have followed this plan for several months now, you will (hopefully) begin to notice the shrinking of your belly fat, increased lean muscle, less food cravings and more energy. Even if you're not able to implement all the changes I've recommended, please know that even small changes are better than doing nothing.

With this book, I want to set you up for sustainable long term weight loss. I know it takes commitment, but you need to set aside all excuses and just stick with the plan.

Because you have eliminated all foods that were holding you back from reaching your weight loss goals, you're improving the health of your gut by adding valuable probiotics and prebiotics to your gut AND you have a more stable and appropriate insulin response throughout the day, you're on your way to permanent, sustainable weight loss.

With this plan, you're allowed to have your favorite foods. You're even allowed to order takeout. And even if you gain a little bit of weight because of the holidays or a party, there's no need to worry because you know that you will lose the weight in just a few days.

I myself have been on this plan for seven years now. Before I started this plan, my routine blood work showed elevated lipids and glucose levels, as well as elevated liver enzymes. My blood pressure slowly went up over the years, and I started to have painful joints. Seven years later, I now have perfect blood pressure and perfect blood work results, and I feel better than ever. I have lost more weight than I could have imagined (and kept it off), and I have greatly improved my BMI.

For the long-term success of this plan and to make sure that you keep your weight off for years to come, I am summarizing the entire plan in the form of a list, so it will be easier to put it all together:

- For breakfast, have an 8-12 Oz. cup of coffee with 5.3 Oz. of FAGE Greek yogurt (recommended 5x per week).
- For lunch, eat 12-16 Oz. of FAGE Greek yogurt sweetened with either fresh fruit or jelly. Have this with an egg or piece of toast. Do this at least 3x per week.
- In between meals, drink plenty of water with a few drops of concentrated lemon juice.
- Have Babybel cheese as a snack 1-2 times per day.
- Use either walnuts, cashews or peanuts as additional snacks. Do not have more than 100 calories each time.
- Drink a full bottle of Kevita probiotic drink at least twice per week.
- Cook a healthy dinner from scratch. Use butter and oil (avocado oil or olive oil). Make sure the protein and fat to carb ratio is high.
- For breads, make sure the bread is made with real, unbleached and unbromated flour (and avoid any breads made with enriched flour).
- Use as much organic foods as possible. When you buy non-organic food products, you run the risk of being exposed to thousands of chemicals, which will interfere with your metabolism.

- Use prebiotics generously (FOS and GOS, see chapter 4): onions, leeks, peas, chickpeas, black beans, bananas.
- Have at least one spicy meal a week. Spicy foods are great for weight loss. Spicy food consumption is correlated with improved cholesterol and lipid levels. Learn how to make curries (for example, Thai curries). While coconut oil is mostly saturated fat, it has been reported to help with weight loss. Coconut milk also contains high amounts of lauric acid, which is naturally present in breast milk. Lauric acid is turned into monolaurin in the body, and is anti-fungal, anti-bacterial and antiviral.
- Add exercise (preferably a combination of aerobic and strength training) to your routine. It will help with your weight loss, as it increases lean muscle and boosts your metabolism.
- Make a meal plan for the week: do your groceries before the start of the work week, and write a grocery list before you go to the store. Doing this will help you stick to your weight loss goals, and reduce the risk of you ordering takeout food. Remember that it only takes 20-30 minutes to prepare a healthy meal from scratch.

The following items are things that should be eliminated from your diet (or at least, greatly reduced):

- Avoid fast food at all costs.
- Avoid trans-fats (partially hydrogenated oils):
  This would require you to read the labels of all
  snacks, cookies and baked goods you buy. For
  this reason, it would be better to buy snacks
  and baked goods at organic grocery stores.
- Avoid high-fructose corn syrup: Try to limit
  high-fructose corn syrup as much as possible,
  as this is one the greatest health risks. It's
  okay to occasionally have a cola if your
  stomach is upset or when you have a
  headache.
- Avoid anything that is labeled low-fat or no-
  fat.
- Avoid anything that is labeled "diet" or "light."
- Do not use any chemical sweeteners (such as
  aspartame, sucralose).
- Do not buy meat, poultry or seafood that is
  non-organic, because you will be exposed to
  hormones and chemicals that will disrupt your
  metabolism.
- Do not buy any pizza that is made with
  enriched flour. Look for pizza restaurants that
  make their pizza dough with real, unbleached,
  bromate-free flour.

- Avoid the temptation to order pizza that comes with breadsticks or any other doughy concoctions that are dipped in a sugary, oily dipping sauce

WITH THIS BOOK, my goal is to give you the knowledge and power to make healthier food choices, to avoid food that is overly processed and contains many chemicals, and to add foods that will give you a healthy gut, increased energy, reduced food cravings and less bloating to your diet.

The importance of a healthy gut and healthy microbiome cannot be overstated. The good bacteria in your gut take components of the (healthy) food you eat that cannot be digested - such as fiber and polyphenols - and transform them into compounds that stimulate hormones such as GLP-1 to control your appetite and metabolism.

Just have the motivation and willpower to stick with this plan, and after a couple of months, this will become second nature. You will never even think about counting calories or points or feel guilty about your food ever again.

REFERENCES

Introduction

- Super Size Me (2004) Documentary. Morgan Spurlock. https://www.imdb.com/title/tt0390521/
- Fit to Fat to Fit (2016 –) TV Series. A&E: https://www.aetv.com/shows/fit-to-fat-to-fit

Chapter 1

- "Products - Data Briefs - Number 313 - July 2018" (https://www.cdc.gov/nchs/products/databriefs/db313.htm) . www.cdc.gov. 7 June 2019.

- https://azdietitians.com/blog/the-history-of-dieting-in-america-2/
- https://www.livestrong.com/article/495400-side-effects-of-bread-water-diet/
- Varady, K. A., Cienfuegos, S., Ezpeleta, M., & Gabel, K. (2021). Cardiometabolic benefits of intermittent fasting. *Annual Review of Nutrition* **41**: 333-361.

Chapter 2

- Holt, S.H.A., Brand Miller, J.C. and Petocz, P. (1997) An Insulin Index of Foods: the Insulin Demand Generated by 1000-kJ Portions of Common Foods. *Am. J. Clin. Nutr.* **66**: 1264-1276.
- Elliott, S.S., Keim, N.L., Stern, J.S., Teff, K. and Havel, P.J. (2002) Fructose, Weight Gain, and the Insulin Resistance Syndrome. *Am. J. Clin. Nutr.* **76**: 911-922.
- Isganaitis, E. and Lustig, R.H. (2005) Fast Food, Central Nervous System Insulin Resistance, and Obesity. *Arterioscler. Thromb. Vasc. Biol.* **25**: 2451-2462.
- Corkey, B.E. (2012) Diabetes: Have We Got It All Wrong? Insulin Hypersecretion and Food Additives: Cause of Obersity and Diabetes? *Diabetes Care* **35**: 2432-2436.

- Willett, W.C. (1998) Dietary Fat and Obesity: an Unconvincing Relation. *Am. J. Clin. Nutr.* **68**: 1149-1150.

- Kavanagh, K., Jones, K.L., Sawyer, J., Kelley, K., Carr, J.J., Wagner, J.D. and Rudel, L.L. (2007) Trans Fat Diet Induces Abdominal Obesity and Changes in Insulin Sensitivity in Monkeys. *Obesity* **15**: 1675-1684.

- Tetri, L.H., Basaranoglu, M., Brunt, E.M., Yerian, L.M. and Neuschwander-Tetri, B.A. (2008) Severe NAFLD with Hepatic Necroinflammatory Changes in Mice Fed Trans Fats and a High Fructose Corn Syrup Equivalent. *Am. J. Physiol. Gastrointest. Liver Physiol.* **295**: G987-G995.

- Karami-Mohajeri, S. and Abdollahi, M. (2011) Toxic influence of organophosphate, carbamate, and organochlorine pesticides on cellular metabolism of lipids, proteins, and carbohydrates: A systematic review. Hum Exp Toxicol. 30: 1119 - 1140.

- Pournourmohammadi, S., Farzami, B., Ostad, S.N., Azizi, E. and Abdollahi, M. (2005) Effects of malathion subchronic exposure on rat skeletal muscle glucose metabolism. *Environ. Tox. Pharm.* **19**: 191-196.

Chapter 3

- Stop counting calories: Put the focus on food quality and healthy lifestyle practices to attain a healthy weight. Harvard Health Publishing. https://www.health.harvard.edu/staying-healthy/stop-counting-calories
- What's with Wheat (2016) – Cyndi O'Meara. Documentary. Director: Justin Brown. https://www.imdb.com/title/tt5882206/

Chapter 5

- Bridge, A., Brown, J. Snider, H., Nasato, M., Ward, W.E., Roy, B.D. and Josse, A.R. (2019) Greek Yogurt and 12 Weeks of Exercise Training on Strength, Muscle Thickness and Body Composition in Lean, Untrained University-Aged Males. *Front. Nutr.* **6**: 55.
- Alajeeli, F., Flayyih, M.T., ALrubaie, A.L. and AK.Khazaal, F. (2016) Effect of Probiotic Consumption in the Level of Peptide YY, Ghrelin Hormone and Body Weight in Iraqi Obese Female. *World J. Pharm. Pharm. Sci.* **5**: 242-248.
- Aoun, A., Darwish, F. and Hamod, N. (2020) The Influence of the Gut Microbiome on Obesity in Adults and the Role of Probiotics, Prebiotics, and Synbiotics for Weight Loss. *Prev. Nutr. Food Sci.* **25**: 113-123.

- https://www.livestrong.com/article/272678-list-of-foods-that-contain-medium-chain-triglycerides/
- What Is MCT Oil? Benefits, Dosage And Side Effects: https://www.forbes.com/health/supplements/what-is-mct-oil/
- Shcherbakova, K., Schwarz, A., Apryatin, S., Karpenko, M. and Trofimov, A. (2022) Supplementation of Regular Diet With Medium-Chain Triglycerides for Procognitive Effects: A Narrative Review. *Front Nutr.* 9: 934497.
- The Science Behind Ozempic Was Wrong (S. Zhang) *The Atlantic*: https://www.theatlantic.com/health/archive/2024/03/ozempic-glp1-weight-loss-brain-gut/677645/
- Your Body Has Its Own Built-In Ozempic. (C. Damian) *Scientific American* (01/25/2024): https://www.scientificamerican.com/article/your-body-has-its-own-built-in-ozempic/
- Ozempic Side Effects: https://www.webmd.com/obesity/ozempic-side-effects
- Aydin, S. (2013) Presence of adropin, nesfatin-1, apelin-12, ghrelins and salusins peptides in the milk, cheese whey and plasma of dairy cows. *Peptides* **43**: 83-87.
- https://www.reverta.com/blog/skin-care/benefits-of-an-alkaline-diet/

Chapter 6

- How Much Lactose is in Yogurt? Get the Facts Here. (2023) D. Miles: https://yogurtnerd.com/how-much-lactose-is-in-yogurt/
- Greek Yogurt For Lactose Intolerance (2021) https://www.usdairy.com/news-articles/lactose-intolerance-and-greek-yogurt
- 6 Dairy Foods That Don't Affect Lactose Intolerance (2016) https://www.prevention.com/food-nutrition/g20511127/dairy-for-lactose-intolerant-people/
- Torres-Gonzales, M. (2020) Does Dairy Lower Your Risk Of Type-2 Diabetes & High Blood Pressure? https://www.usdairy.com/news-articles/does-eating-dairy-lower-risk-type-2-diabetes-high-blood-pressure
- Coconut Yogurt Nutrition Facts and Health Benefits (2023): https://www.verywellfit.com/all-about-coconut-yogurt-4165922
- Forager Project: https://www.foragerproject.com/

Chapter 7

- https://www.ahealthiermichigan.org/2011/07/26/whats-in-your-food-enriched-flour-tops-list-of-unhealty-ingredients/

- Fat: A Documentary – https://www.imdb.com/title/tt8439204/

Chapter 8

- Lee, I. and Buchner, D.M. (2008) The Importance of Walking to Public Health. *Medicine & Science in Sports & Exercise* **40**: S512-S518.
- Penedo, F.J. and Dahn, J.R. (2005). Exercise and well-being: a review of mental and physical health benefits associated with physical activity. *Current opinion in psychiatry* **18**:189-193.

NOTES

1. Not Another Diet...

1. Metabolism is all the biochemical reactions taking place in each cell of the body to produce energy in order to sustain life.

5. The Science Behind This Diet

1. Galactooligosaccharides and Fructose oligo-saccharides (FOS) are a type of sugar linked together in long chains. GOS is derived from cow's milk and FOS can be found in certain fruits and vegetables. Both GOS and FOS are considered prebiotics, which are non-digestible food ingredients that stimulate the growth of good bacteria in the gut such as Bifidobacteria and lactobacilli.

THANK YOU FOR READING 'RESET YOUR GUT DIET'!

I would really like to know what you thought of this book and if the plan helped you in any way.

Every review matters and I would really appreciate your review.

Please go to Amazon and leave your honest review. It'll help fellow readers and will help me create better books.

You can do so by going to your *recent purchases* and select this book *or* by scanning this **QR code** (which will take you to all my books):

Thank you very much!

~Mason Ford

Made in the USA
Monee, IL
12 December 2024

73454506R00075